Vegan Recipes for Bodybuilding

Affordable, Healthy & Delicious Plant-Based Recipes for Athletes who Want to Lose Weight and Build Muscle

Frank Smith

Table of Contents

Vegan Diet and Athletes

Getting your body in shape requires figuring out the kind of diet you can hold indefinitely. This would most commonly be a diet that's affordable, light on your digestion, and in line with your personal beliefsand lifestyle.

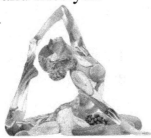

When you add the requirement of achieving athletic results on a vegan diet, you've entered a whole new paradigm of eating that comes down to having a scientifically based and competitive diet that lets you achieve your inner potential to the fullest.

Veganism. You see it all over the place, and lots and lots of people like to talk about it, which, of course, leads to a completely reliable source of information... ha! Wouldn't that be great? But, as humanity kicks in, you start to realize that a lot of these sources are completely untrustworthy.

Now, as more and more people talk about it and more and more opinions get thrown around, mixed in with some fallacies and judgments, combined with some paranoia, and you get yourself a nice, tasty Stew of Ignorance with just a dabble of truth at the bottom, but you can't even see it because of all the stuff floating around on top of it. Don't drink the Stew of Ignorance! Instead, look for real sources who are on the side of the facts (that's me). Through the new chapters, I'll be taking various things out of the Stew of Ignorance until we get to the root of the matter.

The first "ingredient" that mucks up the Stew of Ignorance is myths. Myths, myths, myths. There's about a bazillion of them associated with veganism, but let's knock off each one, one at a time, good and bad, and

give you a real picture of what veganism is actually about. Pour out that Stew of Ignorance!

Myth Number 1: The biggest one is that veganism cannot actually sustain you. You've probably heard this argument before, maybe even toted with a "we aren't rabbits, you know." Funny? Yes. But also completely untrue. Now, there is some merit to this argument, and here it is: if you don't do it right, cutting out meat and dairy products can lead to some deficiencies (like vitamin B, calcium deficiencies, etc.). Here's the thing it all boils down to: if you don't plan, no diet will really work. Before starting such a diet, make sure to be knowledgeable about the potential drawbacks and plan for them, thus destroying Myth Number 1.

Myth Number 2: Veganism makes you healthier than normal diets! It's the exact opposite of Myth Number 1, and it's also just... well, it's just not entirely correct. Yes, various studies have shown that people who are vegans tend to have lower rates of heart disease and cancers and actually just feel better in general. On face value, hooray! Veganism fixes everything! The truth is a bit more complicated: most people who are vegans also practice very healthy lifestyles and, once you remove the figures about meat-eaters who skew the data with terrible health (cigarette smokers, overeaters, etc.), there's about the same low rate between vegans and non-vegans. So, yes, if you are a healthy person and you take care of yourself, you will be better off both in the short and long term.

Myth Number 3: Veganism leads to protein deficiencies. Essential amino acids, which, you guessed it, are essential, serve as the building blocks that make up protein. The body can't make them all, so you have to eat them. Yes, many plant proteins have a pretty low number of essential amino acids (which is protein, basically), which would be terrible if you only ate these foods. However, this can be easily bypassed through the use of other plant-based proteins, like rice and beans, nuts, seeds, legumes, etc. In other words, make sure you're not just having one kind of thing and watch what you eat, and you should have no problems with protein deficiencies. There are a lot of myths about not veganism making people tired, weak, etc., but it all is this same thing: combine foods to properly dodge this. We'll be including some meal plans at the end.

BREAKFAST

1. Stamina Tofu "Omelette"

Ready in Time: 20 minutes | Servings: 2

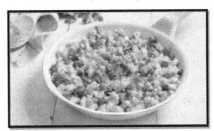

Ingredients

1 Tbsp of olive oil

1 small onion finely chopped 1 large red pepper chopped

1/2 cup white mushrooms halved or sliced 3/4 lb tofu cut into cubes

1 Tbsp nutritional yeast 1 tsp turmeric (for color)

1 tsp of garlic powder

Sea salt and ground black pepper to taste

Instructions

1. Heat oil in a large frying pan over medium-high heat.

2. Sauté onion and red pepper with a pinch of salt

for 2 to 3 minutes.

3.   Add mushrooms and cook until most of the water from the mushroomshas evaporated.

4. Add tofu cubes and all remaining ingredients; stir well.

5.   Cover and cook over medium heat for about 6 to 8 minutes; stiroccasionally.

6. Taste and adjust seasonings.

7. Serve hot.

Nutrition Facts

Percent daily values based on the Reference Daily Intake (RDI) for a2000 calorie diet.

Amount Per Serving

Calories 350.37 | Calories From Fat (60%) 209.61 | Total Fat 24.29g 37%

| Saturated Fat 2.92g 15% |

Cholesterol 0mg 0% | Sodium 24.16mg 1% | Potassium 623.77mg 18% | Total Carbohydrates 17.6g 6% | Fiber 5.28g 21% | Sugar 7g | Protein 21.6g 43%

2. Superelan Vegan Quark Smoothie

Ready in Time: 10 minutes | Servings: 2

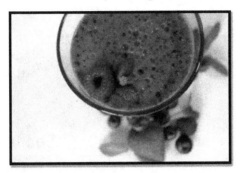

Ingredients

1 frozen banana

3/4 cup frozen berries

1 apple cored and sliced1/3 cup oats

1 scoop vegan protein powder (Soy or Hemp Protein)3/4 cup vegan quark (for example Alpro)

1 1/2 cups almond milk

Instructions

1. Place all ingredients into your fast-speed blender.

2. Blend until smooth and creamy.

3. Serve immediately.

Nutrition Facts

Percent daily values based on the Reference Daily Intake (RDI) for a 2000 calorie diet.

Amount Per Serving

Calories 439.31 | Calories From Fat (27%) 116.9 | Total Fat 13.39g 21% | Saturated Fat 6g 30% |

Cholesterol 33mg 11% | Sodium 114.18mg 5% | Potassium 553.73mg 16% | Total Carbohydrates 76.31g 25% | Fiber 12.2g 49% | Sugar 38.69g | Protein 12g 24%

3. Sweet Potato and Orange Breakfast Bread

Ready in Time: 55 minutes | Servings: 6

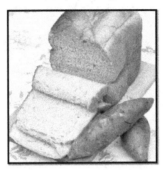

Ingredients

1 large sweet potato (about 12 oz.), peeled and shredded1/2 cup fresh orange juice

1/3 cup water

1/3 cup orange marmalade4 Tbsp canola oil

1Tbsp arrowroot powder 3 cups flour self-rising

1/2 cup sugar tsp baking powder1/4 tsp salt

Instructions

1. Preheat oven to 375 F/180 C.

2. In a small saucepan, cook the shredded sweet potato for 10 min;drain and cool.

3. In a bowl, combine shredder potato

with orange juice, water, orange marmalade, canola oil, and arrowroot powder.

4. In a separate bowl, combine together the flour, sugar, baking powder,and salt.

5. Add the liquid ingredients to the flour mixture and stir just untilcombined.

6. Spoon batter into greased loaf pan and bake for 30-35 minutes.

7. When ready, allow it to cool for 10 minutes.

8. Slice and serve.

Nutrition Facts

Percent daily values based on the Reference Daily Intake (RDI) for a2000 calorie diet.

Amount Per Serving

Calories 481.94 | Calories From Fat (18%) 88.1 | Total Fat 10g15% | Saturated Fat 0.9g 4% | Cholesterol 0mg 0% | Sodium 273.26mg 11% | Potassium 374.4mg 11% | Total Carbohydrates 91.61g 31% | Fiber 2.38g 10% | Sugar 36.31g | Protein 7.58g 15%

4. The Power of Banana & Soya Smoothie

Ready in Time: 10 minutes | Servings: 2

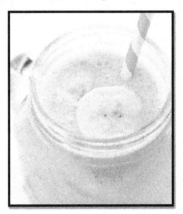

Ingredients

3/4 cup soya milk 2 bananas frozen 1 kiwi fruit sliced

1 Tbsp hemp seeds 1 Tbsp linseed oil

1 scoop vegan protein powder (pea or soy protein)

1 cup fresh spinach

3/4 cup frozen berries thawed (unsweetened)

Instructions

2 Place all ingredients in your blender.

3 Blend for about 45 seconds or until everything is well mixed.

4Serve.

Nutrition Facts

Percent daily values based on the Reference Daily Intake (RDI) for a2000 calorie diet.

Amount Per Serving

Calories 325.59 | Calories From Fat (38%) 122.54 | Total Fat 13.57g 21%

| Saturated Fat 1.61g 8% |

Cholesterol 2.31mg <1% | Sodium 157.75mg 7% | Potassium 916mg 26% | Total Carbohydrates 45.5g 15% | Fiber 7.82g 31% | Sugar 23g | Protein 10g 20%

5. Toasted Tempeh - Vegan Mayo Sandwich

Ready in Time: 10 minutes | Servings: 1

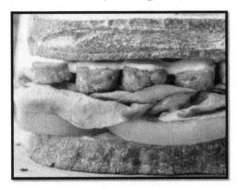

Ingredients

5 slices of bread

2 Tbsp of Vegan Mayo

2 slices of smoky Tempeh cut into strips 1 large tomato sliced

4 leaves of lettuce

Instructions

1. Toast your bread and then spread a layer of Vegan Mayo on oneside of each slice of bread.

2. Layer the Tempeh onto one side of bread and top with tomato slices and lettuce leaves.

3. Cover with the second slice of bread.

4. Enjoy!

Nutrition Facts

Percent daily values based on the Reference Daily Intake (RDI) for a2000 calorie diet.

Amount Per Serving

Calories 535.27 | Calories From Fat (29%) 156.34 | Total Fat 18.69g 29%

| Saturated Fat 2.7g 14% |

Cholesterol 0mg 0% | Sodium 186.34mg 8% | Potassium 913.45mg 26% | Total Carbohydrates 59.41g 20% | Fiber 8.12g 32% | Sugar 3.73g | Protein 39.86g 80%

6. Frozen Berries Vigor Smoothie

Ready in Time: 10 minutes | Servings: 2

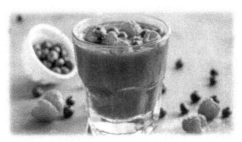

Ingredients

1 1/2 cups almond milk

3/4 cup frozen berries, thawed (any) 1/2 cup fresh spinach leaves chopped1 large banana sliced

3 Tbsp peanut butter 2 Tbsp strained honey

1 scoop vegan protein powder (soy)

Instructions

1. Add all ingredients in your blender, and blend until combined well.

2. Pour your smoothie into the bottle, glass, or Mason jars; cover andkeep refrigerated up to 2 days.

3. Or, pour your smoothie into a freezer-safe

Ziploc bag and freeze up to3 months.

4. Let it defrost in the refrigerator overnight, stir and enjoy!

Nutrition Facts

Percent daily values based on the Reference Daily Intake (RDI) for a2000 calorie diet.

Amount Per Serving

Calories 301 | Calories From Fat (38%) 113.68 | Total Fat 13.52g 21% | Saturated Fat 2.71g 14% | Cholesterol 1.16mg <1% | Sodium 137mg 6% |

Potassium 570.22mg 16% | Total Carbohydrates 41.18g 14% | Fiber 4.72g 19% | Sugar 29.82g | Protein 10g 20%

7. Green Quinoa Breakfast Patties

Ready in Time: 20 minutes | Servings: 4

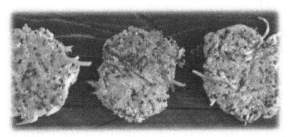

Ingredients

11/2 cup cooked quinoa 1/2 cup shredded carrots

1/2 cup shredded carrots

2Tbsp flaxseed (soaked in 6 Tbsp water) 1/2 cup plain bread crumbs

2 garlic cloves minced1 tsp onion powder

1 tsp garlic powder

2Tbsp fresh parsley finely chopped Salt and ground black pepper to taste

2 Tbsp extra virgin olive oil (plus additional for cooking)Olive oil for frying

Instructions

1. In a large bowl, combine all ingredients until

combined well.

2. Make patties out of the mixture.

3. Heat oil in a non-stick frying skillet.

4. Fry quinoa patties on both sides 2-3 minutes or until crisp.

5. Drain on a plate lined with a paper towel.

6. Keep refrigerated in an airtight container for up to 5 days.

Nutrition Facts

Percent daily values based on the Reference Daily Intake (RDI) for a 2000 calorie diet.

Amount Per Serving

Calories 155.38 | Calories From Fat (12%) 19.11 | Total Fat 2.15g 3% | Saturated Fat 0.18g <1% | Cholesterol 0mg 0% | Sodium 124.87mg 5% | Potassium 265.48mg 8% | Total Carbohydrates 28.8g 10% | Fiber 3.58g 14% | Sugar 2.23g | Protein 5.45g 11%

8. High Protein Chia and Banana Smoothie

Ready in Time: 10 minutes | Servings: 2

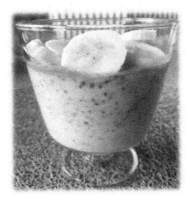

Ingredients

1 1/2 cup of coconut milk (canned)2 Tbsp peanut butter, unsweetened2 Tbsp chia seeds

1 cup celery leaves, finely chopped 1 large banana, sliced

1 scoop vegan protein powder (pea or soy protein)2 Tbsp dark honey strained

Instructions

1. Add all ingredients into high-speed blender; blend until smooth andcombined well.

2. Pour your smoothie into the bottle,

glass, or Mason jars; cover andkeep refrigerated up to 2 days.

3.   Or, pour your smoothie into a freezer-safe Ziploc bag and freeze up to3 months.

4. Let it defrost in the refrigerator overnight, stir and enjoy!

Nutrition Facts

Percent daily values based on the Reference Daily Intake (RDI) for a 2000 calorie diet.

Amount Per Serving

Calories 620,1 | Calories From Fat (66%) 406.92 | Total Fat 48.55g 75% | Saturated Fat 34.23g 171% | Cholesterol 1.16mg <1% | Sodium 129.3mg 5% | Potassium 861.45mg 25% | Total Carbohydrates 44.64g 15% | Fiber 7g28% | Sugar 26.32g | Protein 12.68g 25%

9. Iced Salad and Pineapple Smoothie

Ready in Time: 10 minutes | Servings: 2

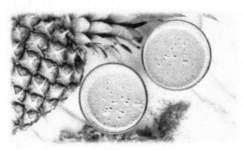

Ingredients

1 1/2 cups soy milk

2Tbsp almond butter (plain, unsalted) 1 small head of lettuce chopped

1 cup raw pineapple chunks

1 large banana, cut into 1-inch pieces

1 scoop vegan protein powder (e.g., chia, soy or hemp)2 Tbsp maple syrup

1 cup iced cubes (optional)

Instructions

1. Combine all ingredients in a blender and blend until smooth.

2. Pour your smoothie into the bottle,

glass, or Mason jars; cover andkeep refrigerated up to 2 days.

3.   Or, pour your smoothie into a freezer-safe Ziploc bag and freeze up to3 months.

4. Let it defrost in the refrigerator overnight, stir and enjoy!

Nutrition Facts

Percent daily values based on the Reference Daily Intake (RDI) for a2000 calorie diet.

Amount Per Serving

Calories 368.7 | Calories From Fat (31%) 114.44 | Total Fat 13.36g 21% |Saturated Fat 1.2g 6% | Cholesterol 1.16mg <1% | Sodium 118.73mg 5% | Potassium 779.15mg 22% | Total Carbohydrates 54g 18% | Fiber 6.15g 25% | Sugar 36.27g | Protein 13.7g 28%

10. **Dried Fruit Energy Bars**

Ready in Time: 10 minutes | Servings: 4

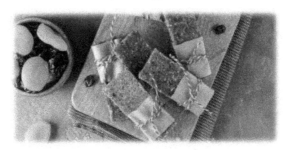

Ingredients

1 cup dried plums chopped1 cup pitted raisins

1 cup dried apricots chopped3 Tbsp lemon juice

1handful of chia seeds2 Tbsp extracted honey

Instructions

1. Add all ingredients in your food processor; process it until getting a smooth mixture.

2. Apply the mixture in a baking sheet, and flat with a spatula; refrigerate the mixture for 2 hours.

3. Cut the mixture into bars.

4. Keep your energy bars tightly covered in the Ziploc bag in therefrigerator or freezer.

Nutrition Facts

Percent daily values based on the Reference Daily Intake (RDI) for a2000 calorie diet.

Amount Per Serving

Calories 280.9 | Calories From Fat (2%) 4.23 | Total Fat 0.51g <1% | Saturated Fat 0.04g <1% | Cholesterol 0mg 0% | Sodium 12.61mg <1% |

Potassium 900.12mg 26% | Total Carbohydrates 74.15g 25% | Fiber 5.9g 24% | Sugar 46.38g | Protein 3.1g 6%

LUNCH

11. Raw Creamy Coconut - Curry Soup

Ready in Time: 10 minutes | Servings: 2

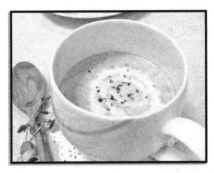

Ingredients

4 Tbsp sesame oil

1/4 cup coconut aminos or soy sauce 1 Tbsp curry powder

1/4 cup fresh lime juice 1/2 cup of tomato sauce 2 Tbsp grated ginger

2 cloves of garlic Salt, to taste

1 cup of canned mushrooms 3 cups coconut milk canned

2 Tbsp fresh chopped mint, to garnish

Instructions

1. Combine ingredients (except coconut milk and mint) in a blender.
2. Blend on high until smooth.
3. Pour in coconut milk, and blend again until combined well.
4. Pour into bowls, sprinkle with fresh mint and serve.
5. Keep refrigerated.

Nutrition Facts

Percent daily values based on the Reference Daily Intake (RDI) for a2000 calorie diet.

Amount Per Serving

Calories 649.42 | Calories From Fat (85%) 550.12 | Total Fat 64.2g 99% | Saturated Fat 36g 180% | Cholesterol 0mg 0% | Sodium 1361mg 48% | Potassium 934.65mg 27% | Total Carbohydrates 18.3g 6% | Fiber 3.16g 13% | Sugar 4.9g | Protein 10.39g 21%

12. Slow-Cooked Navy Bean Soup

Ready in Time: 8 hours | Servings: 8

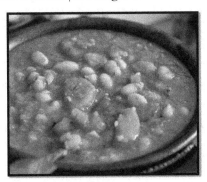

Ingredients

1lb dry navy beans, soaked, rinsed 4 Tbsp olive oil

1/4 cup onion finely diced

2cloves garlic finely chopped2 carrots sliced

1/2 cup tomato sauce (canned)1 tsp mustard

1/2 tsp curry powder6 cups of water

Salt and ground black pepper to taste

Instructions

1. Soak beans overnight.

2. Rinse beans and add in your 6 Quart Slow

Cooker.

3. Add all remaining ingredients and stir well.

4. Cover and cook on LOW for 8 hours.

5. Adjust the salt and pepper to taste.

6. Serve hot.

Nutrition Facts

Percent daily values based on the Reference Daily Intake (RDI) for a2000 calorie diet.

Amount Per Serving

Calories 191.2 | Calories From Fat (4%) 7.6 | Total Fat 0.91g 1% |Saturated Fat 0.11g <1% |

Cholesterol 0mg 0% | Sodium 146.67mg 6% | Potassium 746.42mg 21% | Total Carbohydrates 35.18g 12% | Fiber 13.64g 55% | Sugar 3.85g | Protein 12.15g 24%

13. **Sour Artichoke Hearts with Rice**

Ready in Time: 40 minutes | Servings: 6

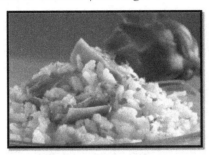

Ingredients

1 cup of olive oil

10 canned artichoke hearts, chopped 2 carrots cut into thin slices

1 cup of long-grain rice 3 cups vegetable broth

2 Tbsp of fresh parsley finely chopped 2 Tbsp fresh dill finely chopped

2 Tbsp apple cider vinegar (optional) Salt and ground pepper to taste

Instructions

1. Heat oil in a large pot over medium-high heat.

2. Add artichokes and sauté for 5 minutes.

3. Add carrots and sprinkle with a pinch of the salt and pepper.

4. Sauté and stir for 2 to 3 minutes.

5. Add rice and stir for one minute.

6. Pour water, and add dill and parsley; stir.

7. Bring to a boil and reduce heat to simmer.

8. Cover and cook for 25 minutes.

9. Taste and adjust seasonings.

10. Pour apple cider vinegar and stir.

11. Serve hot.

Nutrition Facts

Percent daily values based on the Reference Daily Intake (RDI) for a2000 calorie diet.

Amount Per Serving

Calories 445.53 | Calories From Fat (40%) 180.14 | Total Fat 20.41g 31% | Saturated Fat 3g 15% | Cholesterol 1.23mg <1% | Sodium 1025.47mg 43% | Potassium 854.8mg 24% | Total Carbohydrates 58.7g 20% | Fiber 10.55g 42% | Sugar 1.31g | Protein 11g 22%

14. Spring Greens and Rice Stew

Ready in Time: S5 minutes | Servings: 4

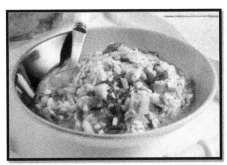

Ingredients

1/3 cup of olive oil

2 cups lettuce salad, chopped

2cups dandelion leaves chopped 1 cup rice short grain

3 cups vegetable broth

1tsp fresh basil finely chopped 2 Tbsp fresh dill chopped

Table salt and ground black pepper to taste

Instructions

1. Heat oil in a large pot over medium-high heat.

2. Sauté lettuce and dandelion leaves for about 4 to 5 minutes.

3. Add rice, cook for one minute; pour rice, and stir.

4. Add in basil, dill, and the salt and ground pepper.

5. Reduce heat to medium-low, cover and cook for about 40 minutes or until all liquid has been absorbed

6. Taste, adjust seasoning, and serve.

Nutrition Facts

Percent daily values based on the Reference Daily Intake (RDI) for a2000 calorie diet.

Amount Per Serving

Calories 470.95 | Calories From Fat (42%) 199.52 | Total Fat 22.66g 35%

| Saturated Fat 3.2g 16% |

Cholesterol 1.85mg <1% | Sodium 1246.8mg 52% | Potassium 499mg 14% | Total Carbohydrates 63.81g 21% | Fiber 7g 28% | Sugar 0.2g | Protein 9g 18%

15. Sweet Potatoes Puree with Almond Milk (SlowCooker)

Ready in Time: 4 hours and 10 minutes | Servings: 4

Ingredients

2 pounds sweet potatoes peeled and cut into small cubes 1/2 cup almond milk

Pink Himalayan salt 2 Tbsp almond butter

1/4 tsp of turmeric powder 1/2 tsp cinnamon

Instructions

1. Rinse potatoes thoroughly to wash away any dirt.

2. Place sweet potato cubes, almond milk, and a pinch of Pink Himalayan salt in your Slow Cooker.

3. Cover and turn to HIGH 2 hours or on LOW for 4 hours.

4. Transfer potatoes in your fast-speed blender.

5. Add all remaining ingredients.

6. Blend until smooth and creamy.

7. If your puree is too thick, add some more almond

milk.

8. Taste and adjust salt to taste.

9. Serve.

Nutrition Facts

Percent daily values based on the Reference Daily Intake (RDI) for a2000 calorie diet.

Amount Per Serving

Calories 244.98 | Calories From Fat (16%) 38.27 | Total Fat 4.57g 7% |Saturated Fat 0.38g 2% |

Cholesterol 0mg 0% | Sodium 184.73mg 8% | Potassium 828mg 24% | Total Carbohydrates 47.31g 16% | Fiber 7.7g 31% | Sugar 9.84g

| Protein 5.94g 12%

16. Hearty and Creamy Corn Chowder

Ready in Time: 20 minutes | Servings: 4

Ingredients

2 cups of frozen whole kernel corn 2 Tbsp chopped onion

1 tsp of grated garlic

2Tbsp finely chopped parsley 4 Tbsp chopped green pepper 1 1/2 cups of vegetable broth 2 Tbsp olive oil

Salt and ground pepper to taste 1 cup of almond milk

2 Tbsp yellow cornmeal

Instructions

1. Add corn, onion, garlic, parsley, green pepper, salt and pepper, vegetable broth, and olive oil in your Instant Pot; stir.

2. Dissolve cornmeal in almond milk and pour in Instant pot; give a goodstir.

3. Lock lid into place and set on the

MANUAL setting high pressure for10 minutes.

4. When the timer beeps, press "Cancel" and carefully flip the QuickRelease valve to let the pressure out.

5. Taste and adjust the salt and pepper to taste; allow to cool completely.

6. Store your chowder in an airtight container, and keep refrigerated up to4 days.

Note: *For quick and easy reheating, store single-serving portions inindividual containers.*

Nutrition Facts

Percent daily values based on the Reference Daily Intake (RDI) for a 2000 calorie diet.

Amount Per Serving

Calories 225.14 | Calories From Fat (39%) 86.92 | Total Fat 9.67g 15% | Saturated Fat 1.2g 6% | Cholesterol 0mg 0% | Sodium 448mg 19% | Potassium 456.18mg 13% | Total Carbohydrates 32.58g 11% | Fiber 4g 16% | Sugar 4.6g | Protein 6.7g 14%

17. **High-protein Quinoa with Celery and Pine Nuts**

Ready in Time: 25 minutes | Servings: 4

Ingredients

4 Tbsp olive oil

2 green onions sliced 1 cup quinoa

1/4 cup pine nuts

4 stalks celery, chopped 3 cups vegetable broth

Sea salt to taste

1/4 cup fresh lemon juice 1/4 tsp cayenne pepper

1/2 tsp ground cumin

2 Tbsp fresh parsley chopped

Instructions

1. Turn on the Instant Pot and press the SAUTÉ button and heat oil.

2. Sauté the green onion with a pinch of salt until soft.

3. Add quinoa and peanuts, and stir for one minute.

4. Add celery, and all remaining ingredients and give a good stir.

5. Lock lid into place and set on the MANUAL setting high pressure for3 minutes.

6. Once the pot beeps finished, use a natural release for 10 minutes.

7. Remove from the pot and allow to cool down.

8. Store in an airtight container in a fridge for up to 5 days.

Nutrition Facts

Percent daily values based on the Reference Daily Intake (RDI) for a 2000 calorie diet.

Amount Per Serving

Calories 470.37 | Calories From Fat (46%) 218.64 | Total Fat 24.6g 38% |Saturated Fat 3.28g 16% | Cholesterol 1.85mg <1% | Sodium 1602.8mg 67% | Potassium 751.2mg 21% | Total Carbohydrates 51.52g 17% | Fiber 6.79g 27% | Sugar 1.73g | Protein 12.56g 25%

18. Instant Fava Bean Soup with Saffron

Ready in Time: 40 minutes | Servings: 4

Ingredients

4 Tbsp olive oil

1 yellow onion finely diced 2 cloves garlic, chopped Kosher salt and freshly ground black pepper, to taste 1 1/2 cups Fava Bean (broad beans) 1 can (11 oz) tomatoes - diced 4 cups vegetable broth

1 tsp crushed saffron threads (or 1/2 tsp of ground turmeric)1 tsp ground cumin

Instructions

1. Turn on the Instant Pot and press the SAUTÉ button; heat oil.

    2. Sauté onion and garlic with the pinch of salt, often stirring, for about 2to 3 minutes.

3. Add fava beans and tomatoes; stir for one minute.

4. Add the vegetable broth, and all remaining ingredients, and stir well.

5. Lock lid into place and set on the MANUAL setting high pressure for30 minutes.

6. Use Quick Release - turn the valve from sealing to venting to releasethe pressure.

7. Allow it to cool completely.

8. Store in an airtight container and keep refrigerated up to 4 to 5 days.

9. You can also freeze your fava beans soup in freezer bags for up to sixmonths.

Nutrition Facts

Percent daily values based on the Reference Daily Intake (RDI) for a 2000 calorie diet.

Amount Per Serving

Calories 331.33 | Calories From Fat (46%) 153.58 | Total Fat 17.37g 27%

| Saturated Fat 2.72g 14% | Cholesterol 2.15mg <1% | Sodium 1548.13mg 65% | Potassium 695.25mg 20% | Total Carbohydrates 37.2g 13% | Fiber 4.14g 17% | Sugar 3.17g | Protein 10g 20%

19. **Instant Lentils Bolognese**

Ready in Time: S5 minutes | Servings: 5

Ingredients

4 Tbsp olive oil1 large onion

2 cloves garlic finely chopped Salt and ground pepper to taste

2 cup of red lentils1 carrot sliced

1 can (15 oz) peeled tomatoes4 cups of vegetable broth

1 Tbsp Italian seasoning

Instructions

1. Press the SAUTÉ button on your Instant Pot, and add oil.

2. Sauté the onion and garlic with a pinch of salt until soft or for about 3minutes.

3. Add lentils and stir for a further one minute.

4. Add carrots and tomatoes, and stir for one minute.

5. Add broth and Italian seasoning.

6. Lock lid into place and set on the MANUAL setting high pressure for15 minutes.

7.   Once cooking completes, let the pressure valve release naturally (about 10 minutes), and quick-release remaining pressure.

8. Taste and adjust seasonings; allow it to cool completely.

9.   Store in a covered glass or airtight container in the fridge for up to 4days.

10. Or, you can freeze your lentils for two months.

Nutrition Facts

Percent daily values based on the Reference Daily Intake (RDI) for a 2000 calorie diet.

Amount Per Serving

Calories 522.2 | Calories From Fat (25%) 131.53 | Total Fat 14.85g 23% | Saturated Fat 2.34g 12% | Cholesterol 2mg <1% | Sodium 1372.65mg 57% | Potassium 1206.23mg 34% | Total Carbohydrates 73.36g 24% | Fiber 27.37g 109% | Sugar 4.28g | Protein 25.42g 51%

20. **Jasmine Rice and Peas Risotto**

Ready in Time: 25 minutes | Servings: 4

Ingredients

4 Tbsp olive oil

1 medium onion finely diced 2 cloves garlic minced

Salt and ground black pepper to taste

1 1/2 cups dry jasmine rice (or long grain rice) 1/2 cup of green peas

1 bay leaf

2cups of vegetable broth2 cups of water

Instructions

1. Press the SAUTÉ button on your Instant Pot.

   2. When the word "hot" appears on display, add the oil and sauté the onion and garlic with a pinch of salt for about 5 minutes; stir frequently.

3. Add the jasmine rice and stir for one minute.

4. Add green peas, and all remaining ingredients and

stir well.

5.   Lock lid into place and set on the RICE setting high pressure for 6minutes.

6.   When the timer beeps, press "Cancel" and use a Natural release for 10to 15 minutes.

7. Taste and adjust the salt and pepper to taste.

8. Allow cooling completely.

9.   Store your risotto in an airtight container, and keep refrigerated up to 4to 5 days.

Nutrition Facts

Percent daily values based on the Reference Daily Intake (RDI) for a 2000 calorie diet.

Amount Per Serving

Calories 421 | Calories From Fat (34%) 144.5 | Total Fat 16.58g 26% | Saturated Fat 2.1g 11% | Cholesterol 0mg 0% | Sodium 59.4mg 2% | Potassium 181mg 5% | Total Carbohydrates 67.1g 22% | Fiber 5.81g 23% | Sugar 2.3g | Protein 8.21g 16%

DINNER

21. Oven-baked Smoked Lentil 'Burgers'

Ready in Time: 1 hour and 20 minutes | Servings: 6

Ingredients

1 1/2 cups dried lentils3 cups of water

Salt and ground black pepper to taste2 Tbsp olive oil

1 onion finely diced

2 cloves minced garlic

1 cup button mushrooms sliced 2 Tbsp tomato paste

1/2 tsp fresh basil finely chopped 1 cup chopped almonds 3 tsp balsamic vinegar 3 Tbsp coconut aminos1 tsp liquid smoke

3/4 cup silken tofu soft3/4 cup corn starch

Instructions

1.   Cook lentils in salted water until tender

or for about 30-35 minutes; rinse, drain, and set aside.

2. Heat oil in a frying skillet and sauté onion, garlic and mushrooms for 4 to 5 minutes; stir occasionally.

3. Stir in the tomato paste, salt, basil, salt, and black pepper; cook for 2 to3 minutes.

4. Stir in almonds, vinegar, coconut aminos, liquid smoke, and lentils.

5. Remove from heat and stir in blended tofu and corn starch.

6. Keep stirring until all ingredients combined well.

7. Form mixture into patties and refrigerate for an hour.

8. Preheat oven to 350 F.

9. Line a baking dish with parchment paper and arrange patties on thepan.

10. Bake for 20 to 25 minutes.

11. Serve hot with buns, green salad, tomato sauce...etc.

Nutrition Facts

Percent daily values based on the Reference Daily Intake (RDI) for a 2000 calorie diet.

Amount Per Serving

Calories 439.12 | Calories From Fat (34%) 148.97 | Total Fat 17.48g 27% | Saturated Fat 1.71g 9% |

Cholesterol 0mg 0% | Sodium 330mg 14% | Potassium 805.8mg 23% | Total Carbohydrates 53.72g 18% | Fiber 18.19g 73% | Sugar 4.6g | Protein 19.37g 39%

22. **Powerful Spinach and Mustard Leaves Puree**

Ready in Time: 50 minutes | Servings: 4

Ingredients

2 Tbsp almond butter 1 onion finely diced 2 Tbsp minced garlic

1 tsp salt and black pepper (or to taste) 1 lb mustard leaves, cleaned rinsed

1 lb frozen spinach thawed 1 tsp coriander

1 tsp ground cumin 1/2 cup almond milk

Instructions

1. Press the SAUTÉ button on your Instant Pot and heat the almondbutter.

2. Sauté onion, garlic, and a pinch of salt for 2-3 minutes; stiroccasionally.

3. Add spinach and the mustard greens and stir for a minute or two.

4. Season with the salt and pepper, coriander, and cumin; give a good stir.

5. Lock lid into place and set on the MANUAL setting for 15 minutes.

6. Use Quick Release - turn the valve from sealing to venting to releasethe pressure.

7. Transfer mixture to a blender, add almond milk and blend untilsmooth.

8. Taste and adjust seasonings.

9. Serve.

Nutrition Facts

Percent daily values based on the Reference Daily Intake (RDI) for a2000 calorie diet.

Amount Per Serving

Calories 180.53 | Calories From Fat (46%) 82.69 | Total Fat 10g 15% |Saturated Fat 0.65g 3% |Cholesterol 0mg 0% | Sodium 1519.12mg 63% | Potassium 846mg 24% | Total Carbohydrates 17.46g 6% | Fiber 6.92g 28% | Sugar 2.13g | Protein 10.65g 21%

23. Quinoa and Rice Stuffed Peppers (oven-baked)

Ready in Time: S5 minutes | Servings: 8

Ingredients

3/4 cup long-grain rice

8 bell peppers (any color)2 Tbsp olive oil

1 onion finely diced cloves chopped garlic

1 can (11 oz) crushed tomatoes

1 tsp cumin 1 tsp coriander

4 Tbsp ground walnuts2 cups cooked quinoa

4 Tbsp chopped parsley

Salt and ground black pepper to taste

Instructions

1. Preheat oven to 400 F/200 C.

2. Boil rice and drain in a colander.

3. Cut the top stem section of the pepper off, remove the remaining pith and seeds, rinse peppers. Heat oil in a large frying skillet, and sauté onion and garlic until soft.

4. Add tomatoes, cumin, ground almonds, salt, pepper, and coriander; stir well and simmer for 2 minutes stirring constantly.

5. Remove from the heat and add the rice, quinoa, and parsley; stir well.

6. Taste and adjust salt and pepper.

7. Fill the peppers with a mixture, and place peppers cut side-up in a baking dish; drizzle with little oil. Bake for 15 minutes. Serve warm.

Nutrition Facts

Percent daily values based on the Reference Daily Intake (RDI) for a2000 calorie diet.

Amount Per Serving

Calories 335.69 | Calories From Fat (25%) 83.63 | Total Fat 9.58g 15% |Saturated Fat 1.2g 5% |Cholesterol 0mg 0% | Sodium 66.14mg 3% | Potassium 678.73mg 19% | Total Carbohydrates 55.13g 18% | Fiber 8.25g 33% | Sugar 7.8g | Protein 9.8g 20%

24. Quinoa and Lentils with Crushed Tomato

Ready in Time: S5 minutes | Servings: 4

Ingredients

4 Tbsp olive oil

1 medium onion, diced2 garlic clove, minced

Salt and ground black pepper to taste1 can (15 oz) tomatoes crushed

1 cup vegetable broth

1/2 cup quinoa, washed and drained1 cup cooked lentils

1 tsp chili powder1 tsp cumin

Instructions

1.   Heat oil in a pot and sauté the onion and garlic with the pinch of saltuntil soft.

2.   Pour reserved tomatoes and vegetable broth, bring to boil, and stirwell.

3. Stir in the quinoa, cover and cook for 15 minutes; stir occasionally.

4. Add in lentils, chili powder, and cumin; cook for further 5 minutes.

5. Taste and adjust seasonings.

6. Serve immediately.

7. Keep refrigerated in a covered container for 4 - 5 days.

Nutrition Facts

Percent daily values based on the Reference Daily Intake (RDI) for a2000 calorie diet.

Amount Per Serving

Calories 397.45 | Calories From Fat (35%) 138.18 | Total Fat 15.61g 24%

| Saturated Fat 2.14g 11% |

Cholesterol 0mg 0% | Sodium 343.8mg 14% | Potassium 738.51mg21% | Total Carbohydrates 49.32g 16% | Fiber 16.7g 68% | Sugar2.35g | Protein 16.6g 33%

25. **Silk Tofu Penne with Spinach**

Ready in Time: 25 minutes | Servings: 4

Ingredients

1 lb penne, uncooked

12 oz of frozen spinach, thawed 1 cup silken tofu mashed

1/2 cup soy milk (unsweetened) 1/2 cup vegetable broth

1 Tbsp white wine vinegar 1/2 tsp Italian seasoning

Salt and ground pepper to taste

Instructions

1. Cook penne pasta according to package directions; rinse anddrain in a colander.

2. Drain spinach well, squeezing out excess liquid.

3. Place spinach with all remaining ingredients in a blender and beat untilsmooth.

4. Pour the spinach mixture over pasta.

5. Taste and adjust the salt and pepper.

6. Store pasta in an airtight container in the refrigerator for 3 to 5 days.

Nutrition Facts

Percent daily values based on the Reference Daily Intake (RDI) for a2000 calorie diet.

Amount Per Serving

Calories 492.8 | Calories From Fat (5%) 27.06 | Total Fat 3.07g 5% |Saturated Fat 0.38g 2% |

Cholesterol 0.31mg <1% | Sodium 491.22mg 20% | Potassium 433mg 12% | Total Carbohydrates 92.45g 31% | Fiber 7.8g 31% | Sugar 1.21g | Protein 21.61g 43%

26. **Gigante Beans and Tomatoes Stew**

Ready in Time: 1 hour and 10 minutes | Servings: 6

Ingredients

3/4 lbs Gigante Beans soaked overnight1/2 cup of olive oil large onion, finely chopped 3 cloves garlic finely sliced salt and freshly ground pepper

3/4 lb grated tomatoes or canned peeled tomatoes

1/2 bunch of parsley, finely chopped

1/2 Tbsp fresh thyme 1/2 tsp crushed red pepper flakes2 cups of vegetable broth cups of water

Instructions

1. Soak the Gigante beans covered in a warm place.

2. Press the SAUTÉ button on your Instant Pot and heat the oil. Sauté the onion and garlic with a pinch of salt and pepper until soft.

3. Add grated tomatoes and soaked beans; stir for two minutes.

4. Add parsley, thyme, and red flakes; stir.

5. Add water and broth, and give a good stir.

6. Lock lid into place and set on the MANUAL setting high pressure for50 minutes.

7. Once the pot beeps finished, use the Naturally release for 10 minutes and quick-release remaining pressure.

8. Taste and adjust the salt and pepper to taste.

9. Store in an airtight container, and keep refrigerated up to 4 to 5 daysor keep frozen in a freezer-bags up to 4 to 5 months.

Nutrition Facts

Percent daily values based on the Reference Daily Intake (RDI) for a2000 calorie diet.

Amount Per Serving

Calories 428,43 | Calories From Fat (41%) 175,92 | Total Fat 19.92g 31% | Saturated Fat 2.93g 15% | Cholesterol 0.82mg <1% | Sodium 558.12mg 23% | Potassium 1349.68mg 39% | Total Carbohydrates 48.61g 16% | Fiber 11g 44% | Sugar 3.61g | Protein 16.53g 34%

27. **Greek Ratatouille**

Ready in Time: 25 minutes | Servings: 4

Ingredients

3/4 of olive oil

1 onion finely diced

2cloves garlic finely sliced Salt and ground pepper to taste2 potatoes cut into cubes

1 eggplant cut into cubes 1 lb zucchini cut into rings

1 pepper (red-green) sliced

2Tbs fresh chopped mint, basil, and parsley1 can (11 oz) of crushed tomatoes

1 tsp tomato paste1 cup of water

1 vegetable bouillon cube of 1 cup of vegetable broth

Instructions

1. Pour oil to the inner stainless steel pot in the Instant Pot.

2. Turn on the Instant Pot and press the SAUTÉ button.

3. When the word "HOT" appears on display, sauté the onion and garlicwith a pinch of the salt and pepper for about 3 to 4 minutes.

4. Add potato and eggplant cubes and stir for one minute.

5. Add zucchini and pepper and stir for one minute.

6. Add fresh chopped mint, basil and parsley, and stir well.

7. Add crushed tomatoes, tomato paste, water, and vegetable bouilloncube or one cup of vegetable broth; stir well.

8. Lock lid into place and set on the MANUAL setting high pressure for12 minutes.

9. Use Quick Release - turn the valve from sealing to venting to releasethe pressure.

10. Stir, taste and adjust the salt and pepper to taste.

11. Store in an airtight container in the fridge for up to 4 days.

Nutrition Facts

Percent daily values based on the Reference

Daily Intake (RDI) for a 2000 calorie diet.

Amount Per Serving

Calories 184.64 | Calories From Fat (35%) 65.1 | Total Fat 7.39g 11% | Saturated Fat 1.1g 5% | Cholesterol 0mg 0% | Sodium 190.2mg 8% | Potassium 961.61mg 27% | Total Carbohydrates 27.4g 9% | Fiber 4.9g 20% | Sugar 7.73g | Protein 4.61g 9%

28. **Mediterranean Pie Stuffed with Black Olives**

Ready in Time: 1 hour and 5 minutes | Servings: 10

Ingredients

For dough

3 1/2 cup of flour all-purposes2 1 tsp baking soda

1 1/3 cups of olive oil

1 1/4 cups of orange juice

For stuffing

4 Tbsp of olive oil

2large onions, finely chopped 3 cups of black olives pitted

3tsp of fresh mint finely chopped 1 tsp sesame seeds toasted

1 tsp cumin seeds, crushed

Instructions

1. Preheat oven to 360 F.
2. Prepare and grease a round baking pan.
3. Combine the flour with the baking powder in a large bowl.

4. Whisk the olive oil and orange juice into a large bowl; stir well.

5. Combine the flour with the oil mixture, and knead well until get a smooth and light dough.

6. Divide dough into 2 sheets.

7. Heat the oil in a frying skillet and sauté onion until translucent; add olives and fresh chopped mint.

8. Stir and cook for about 3 minutes.

9. Place one sheet of dough into a prepared baking dish and spread the filling; sprinkle with sesame seeds and cumin.

10. Cover the mixture with the second sheet and gently chop the pie into pieces.

11. Bake for 45 minutes or until golden brown.

12. Remove from the oven, and let it sit until cool down completely.

13. Store in an airtight container and keep refrigerated up to 4 to 5 days or freeze your pie

for up to one month.

Nutrition Facts

Percent daily values based on the Reference Daily Intake (RDI) for a 2000 calorie diet.

Amount Per Serving

Calories 426.55 | Calories From Fat (55%) 232.85 | Total Fat 26.53g 41%

| Saturated Fat 3.64g 18% | Cholesterol 0mg 0% | Sodium 475.5mg 20% | Potassium 169.7mg 5% | Total Carbohydrates 42.64g 14% | Fiber 3.14g 13% | Sugar 4.28g | Protein 5.43g 11%

29. Penne with Lemony Asparagus

Ready in Time: S0 minutes | Servings: 2

Ingredients

8 oz pasta (of your preference) 2 cups sliced asparagus

4 Tbs olive oil

1/2 cup green onions, chopped 2 cloves garlic minced

2 Tbsp fresh lemon juice2 tsp lemon rind

salt and ground black pepper to taste

Instructions

1. Cook pasta according to package directions.

    2. Add asparagus to pasta during the last 3 minutes of cooking time;drain.

3. Heat oil in a large frying skillet over medium-high heat.

    4. Sauté green onions and garlic with a pinch of salt for about 4 to 5minutes.

    5. Add pasta, asparagus, lemon juice, lemon

rind, and the salt and pepperto taste.

6. Stir and cook for two minutes.

7. Taste and adjust the salt.

8. Store pasta in an airtight container in the fridge for up to 4 days.

Nutrition Facts

Percent daily values based on the Reference Daily Intake (RDI) for a2000 calorie diet.

Amount Per Serving

Calories 703.14 | Calories From Fat (37%) 257.34 | Total Fat 29g 45%

| Saturated Fat 4.05g 20% | Cholesterol 0mg 0% | Sodium 161.21mg 7% | Potassium 556.6mg 16% | Total Carbohydrates 94.12g 31% | Fiber 6.31g 25% | Sugar 3.64g | Protein 18.16g 36%

SNACKS

30. Mediterranean Marinated Olives

Preparation Time: 10 minutes | Servings: 2

Ingredients

24 large olives, black, green, Kalamata 1/2 cup extra-virgin olive oil

4 cloves garlic, thinly sliced 2 Tbsp fresh lemon juice

2 tsp coriander seeds, crushed 1/2 tsp crushed red pepper

1 tsp dried thyme

1 tsp dried rosemary, crushed Salt and ground pepper to taste

Instructions

1. Place olives and all remaining ingredients in a large container or bag, and shake to combine well.

2. Cover and refrigerate to marinate overnight.

3. Serve.

4. Keep refrigerated.

Nutrition Facts

Percent daily values based on the Reference Daily Intake (RDI) for a2000 calorie diet.

Amount Per Serving

Calories 573.31 | Calories From Fat (94%) 540 | Total Fat 61.36g 94% |Saturated Fat 8.41g 42% |

Cholesterol 0mg 0% | Sodium 578.6mg 24% | Potassium 76.4mg 2% | Total Carbohydrates 8.6g 3% |

Fiber 3.33g 13% | Sugar 0.46g | Protein 1.18g 2%

31. **Nut Butter & Dates Granola**

Ready in Time: 1 hour | Servings: 8

Ingredients

3 cups rolled oats

2 cups dates, pitted and chopped 1 cup flaked or shredded coconut1/2 cup wheat germ

1/4 cup soy milk powder 1/2 cup almonds chopped3/4 cup honey strained

1/2 cup almond butter (plain, unsalted) softened1/4 cup peanut butter softened

Instructions

1. Preheat oven to 300F.

2. Add all ingredients into a food processor and pulse until roughlycombined.

3. Spread mixture evenly into greased 10 x 15-inch baking pan.

4. Bake for 45 to 55 minutes.

5. Stir mixture several times during baking.

6. Remove from the oven and cool completely.

7. Store in a covered glass jar.

Nutrition Facts

Percent daily values based on the Reference Daily Intake (RDI) for a2000 calorie diet.

Amount Per Serving

Calories 586 | Calories From Fat (30%) 177.61 | Total Fat 21.22g 33% | Saturated Fat 4.64g 23% |

Cholesterol 0mg 0% | Sodium 72.47mg 3% | Potassium 734.14mg 21% | Total Carbohydrates 94.85g 32% | Fiber 11.41g 46% | Sugar 56g | Protein 13.9g 28%

32. **Oven-baked** **Caramelize** **Plantains**

Ready in Time: S0 minutes | Servings: 4

Ingredients

4 medium plantains, peeled and sliced 2 Tbsp fresh orange juice

4 Tbsp brown sugar or to taste 1 Tbsp grated orange zest

4 Tbsp coconut butter, melted

Instructions

1. Preheat oven to 360 F/180 C.
2. Place plantain slices in a heatproof dish.
     3. Pour the orange juice over plantains, and then sprinkle with brown sugar and grated orange zest.
4. Melt coconut butter and pour evenly over plantains.
5. Cover with foil and bake for 15 to 17 minutes.
6. Serve warm or cold with honey or maple syrup.

Nutrition Facts

Percent daily values based on the Reference Daily Intake (RDI) for a2000 calorie diet.

Amount Per Serving

Calories 350.51 | Calories From Fat (4%) 14 | Total Fat 1.64g 3% |Saturated Fat 0.83g 4% |

Cholesterol 2.15mg <1% | Sodium 13.04mg <1% | Potassium 1139.42mg 33% | Total Carbohydrates 85.34g 28% | Fiber 5.36g 21% | Sugar 46g | Protein 3g 6%

33. **Powerful Peas & Lentils Dip**

Ready in Time: 10 minutes | Servings: 4

Ingredients

4 cups frozen peas

2 cup green lentils cooked 1 piece of grated ginger 1/2 cup fresh basil chopped 1 cup ground almonds Juice of 1/2 lime

Pinch of salt

4 Tbsp sesame oil 1/4 cup Sesame seeds

Instructions

1. Place all ingredients in a food processor or in a blender.

2. Blend until all ingredients combined well.

3. Keep refrigerated in an airtight container up to 4 days.

Nutrition Facts

Percent daily values based on the Reference Daily Intake (RDI) for a2000 calorie diet.

Amount Per Serving

Calories 561.49 | Calories From Fat (51%) 287.84 | Total Fat 33.64g 52% | Saturated Fat 4g 20% |

Cholesterol 0mg 0% | Sodium 149.13mg 6% | Potassium 825.81mg 24% | Total Carbohydrates 47g 16% | Fiber 18.61g 74% | Sugar 9.48g | Protein 23.8g 48%

34. Protein "Raffaello" Candies

Ready in Time: 15 minutes | Servings: 12

Ingredients

1 1/2 cups desiccated coconut flakes 1/2 cup coconut butter softened

4 Tbsp coconut milk canned

4 Tbs coconut palm sugar (or granulated sugar)1 tsp pure vanilla extract

1 Tbsp vegan protein powder (pea or soy) 15 whole almonds

Instructions

1. Put 1 cup of desiccated coconut flakes, and all remaining ingredients in the blender (except almonds), and blend until soft.

2. If your dough is too thick, add some coconut milk.

3. In a bowl, add remaining coconut flakes.

4. Coat every almond in one tablespoon of mixture and roll into a ball.

5. Roll each ball in coconut flakes.

6. Chill in the fridge for several hours.

Nutrition Facts

Percent daily values based on the Reference Daily Intake (RDI) for a2000 calorie diet.

Amount Per Serving

Calories 212.41 | Calories From Fat (81%) 171.5 | Total Fat 20.32g 31% |Saturated Fat 15g 75% |

Cholesterol 0.15mg <1% | Sodium 8mg <1% | Potassium 137.36mg 4% | Total Carbohydrates 7.62g 3% | Fiber 2.5g 12% | Sugar 3.29g | Protein 3g 6%

35. **Oat Biscuits with Seeds**

Ready in Time: S0 minutes | Yield: 16 biscuits | Servings: 4

Ingredients

4 Tbsp coconut butter melted1/2 cup of oatmeal

1/2 cup almond flour1 tsp baking soda

2 Tbsp sesame seeds2 tsp poppy seeds

5 to 6 Tbsp of warm water

Instructions

1. Heat oven to 360 F.

2. Grease a large baking sheet and sprinkle with the flour; set aside.

3. Add all ingredients into a bowl, and stir well combine to make a firmdough.

4. Transfer dough onto a lightly floured surface and roll out until gettinga thick dough.

5. Cut into small squares and place onto a prepared baking sheet.

6. Bake for about 13 to15 minutes.

7. Remove from the oven, and allow to cool completely.

8.   Place biscuits in an airtight container and keep at room temperature upto 2 weeks.

Nutrition Facts

Percent daily values based on the Reference Daily Intake (RDI) for a 2000 calorie diet.

Amount Per Serving

Calories 229.21 | Calories From Fat (68%) 155.1 | Total Fat 17.76g 27% | Saturated Fat 12.38g 62% | Cholesterol 0mg 0% | Sodium 317.12mg 13% | Potassium 115.24mg 3% | Total Carbohydrates 14.37g 5% | Fiber 2.87g 11% | Sugar 0.06g | Protein 4.34g 9%

36. Olive Crackers

Preparation Time: S5 minutes | Servings: 16

Ingredients

3/4 cup of flour all-purposes1 tsp yeast

pinch of salt

1/2 cup of olive oil 1 tsp garlic powder 1/2 cup almond milk

12 black olives finely chopped1 tsp oregano

2 Tbsp nut cheese (any) crumbled

Instructions

1. Preheat oven to 400 F.

2. Line a baking sheet with parchment paper; set aside.

3. Combine flour, yeast, salt, garlic powder, and almond milk.

4. Stir with a wooden spoon until combined well.

5. Knead the dough by hand until smooth.

6. Form the dough into a ball, wrap in cling film and refrigerate for 2hours.

7. Take the dough out, fold chopped

olives, oregano, and nut cheese;knead lightly.

8. Dust the working surface with flour and roll the dough.

9. Cut the crackers, and arrange on a prepared baking sheet.

10. Bake for 12 to 15 minutes or until golden brown.

11. Store in a sealed container and keep refrigerated for one week.

Nutrition Facts

Percent daily values based on the Reference Daily Intake (RDI) for a 2000 calorie diet.

Amount Per Serving

Calories 138.3 | Calories From Fat (75%) 103.18 | Total Fat 11.86g 18% | Saturated Fat 1.57g 8% | Cholesterol 0mg 0% | Sodium 373.41mg 16% | Potassium 23.3mg <1% | Total Carbohydrates 7.63g 3% | Fiber 1.76g 7% | Sugar 0.08g | Protein 1.27g 3%

37. **Oven-baked Kale-Cashews Chips**

Inactive Time: 1 hour | Total Time: 2 hours and 40 minutes | Servings: 6

Instructions

1 cup cashews chopped (soaked)

1 lb fresh kale leaves cut in large pieces 3 Tbsp lemon juice Tbsp water

2cloves garlic minced1/3 cup of olive oil

1 tsp red sweet paprikaPinch of salt

Instructions

1. Soak the cashews in water for at least one hour; drain.

2. Preheat the oven to 200 F.

3. Line a large baking sheet with a foil or parchment paper; set aside.Wash and rinse kale thoroughly and tear the kale in large pieces.

4. Add drained cashews with lemon juice, water, garlic, olive oil, and red paprika in a blender. Blend on HIGH until smooth and combined well.

5. In a large bowl, toss the cashews sauce with kale to combine well

6. Spread the kale leaves evenly on a prepared baking sheet.

7. Bake for 2 1/2 hours, flipping twice.

8. Remove kale chips and allow them to cool down completely.

9. Place kale chips in a zip lock bag and keep refrigerated.

Nutrition Facts

Percent daily values based on the Reference Daily Intake (RDI) for a 2000 calorie diet.

Amount Per Serving

Calories 200.46 | Calories From Fat (73%) 145.57 | Total Fat 16.71g 26%

| Saturated Fat 2.55g 13% | Cholesterol 0mg 0% | Sodium 133.25mg 6% | Potassium 422.7mg 12% | Total Carbohydrates 11.2g 4% | Fiber 2g 8% | Sugar 1.13g | Protein 4.2g 8%

38. **Pesto Dip with Nuts**

Ready in Time: 10 minutes | Servings: 4

Ingredients

1 cup fresh basil leaves, chopped

2cups zucchini, peeled and chopped 2 cloves garlic minced 1 cup walnuts soaked 1 cup lemon juice from 2 lemons, freshly squeezed

Instructions

1. Add all ingredients in a high-speed blender; blend until completelysmooth.

2. Taste and adjust seasonings to taste.

3. Keep refrigerated in a sealed glass jar for up to one week.

Nutrition Facts

Percent daily values based on the Reference Daily Intake (RDI) for a2000 calorie diet.

Amount Per Serving

Calories 67.38 | Calories From Fat (64%) 43 | Total Fat 5.14g 8% | Saturated Fat 0.52g 3% | Cholesterol 0mg 0% | Sodium 6.38mg <1% |

SWEETS/DESSERTS

39. Dark Honey Hazelnut Cookies

Ready in Time: S0 minutes | Servings: 12

Ingredients

1 Tbsp olive oil

1/2 cup ground hazelnuts1/2 tsp baking soda

1 1/2 cups of hazelnut flour 2 Tbsp of coconut flour 1/2 tsp cinnamonPinch of salt

1 medium banana mashed 2 Tbsp coconut oil melted 4 Tbsp dark honey strained 1 tsp of pure vanilla extract

Instructions

1. Preheat oven to 340 F.

2. Grease a baking sheet with olive oil; set aside.

3. Combine together ground hazelnuts, baking soda, hazelnut flour, coconut flour, cinnamon, and salt in a bowl.

4. In a separate bowl, whisk mashed banana,

coconut oil, dark honey, andvanilla extract.

5. Combine the hazelnut flour mixture with the egg mixture; beatwith the electric mixer until smooth and combined well.

6. Shape the dough into 12 balls; place in a prepared baking sheet. Bake for about 17 to 18 minutes.

7. Remove from the oven; leave to cool for 15 minutes and serve.

8. Keep stored in a covered container.

Nutrition Facts

Percent daily values based on the Reference Daily Intake (RDI) for a2000 calorie diet.

Amount Per Serving

Calories 99.65 | Calories From Fat (56%) 55.45 | Total Fat 6.5g 10% |Saturated Fat 2.36g 12% | Cholesterol 0mg 0% | Sodium 508.6mg 21% | Potassium 78.48mg 2% | Total Carbohydrates 10.15g 3% | Fiber 1g 4% | Sugar 7.13g | Protein 1.8g 4%

40. **Energy Dried Figs Brownies**

Ready in Time: 15 minutes | Servings: 4

Ingredients

1 cup dried figs finely chopped 2 Tbsp cocoa powder

1 cup almonds chopped2 Tbsp extracted honey

1 scoop protein powder (pea or soy) 2 Tbsp of water

Instructions

1. Add all ingredients in a food processor.

2. Process until combined well.

3. Transfer mixture into a bowl, and knead with your hands.

    4. Lay a mixture on working surface and roll dough into about 1/3 of aninch thick sheet.

5. Cut the mixture into the square.

6. Refrigerate for one hour before serving.

Nutrition Facts

Percent daily values based on the Reference Daily Intake (RDI) for a2000 calorie diet.

Amount Per Serving

Calories 347.41 | Calories From Fat (46%) 160.54 | Total Fat 19.14g 29% | Saturated Fat 1.7g 9% |

Cholesterol 0.58mg <1% | Sodium 15mg <1% | Potassium 576.7mg 16% | Total Carbohydrates 41.83g 14% | Fiber 8.52g 34% | Sugar 28.38g | Protein 10.31g 21%

CPSIA information can be obtained
at www.ICGtesting.com
Printed in the USA
BVHW040319120521
607043BV00001B/162

9 781802 890785